I0425586

ACTIVE WALKING MEDITATION FOR BEGINNERS

ELIMINATES ANXIETY, INCREASES YOUR SELF-ESTEEM, IMPROVES YOUR RELAXATION BEFORE GOING TO SLEEP, SPIRITUAL ABUNDANCE

Jorge O. Chiesa

Copyright 2019 © Jorge O. Chiesa

All rights reserved. No part of this publication may be reproduced or distributed in any form or by any means, electronic or mechanical, including photocopying, recording, or by any information storage or retrieval system, without the prior written permission of the authors.

First Edition

Table of Contents

Introduction: Meditation while walking

In this method of meditation, you will be able to acquire not only the basic knowledge of walking meditation, but an extreme power to elevate yourself and your inner experience and feeling beyond tradition and definition.

Walking meditation is generally understood as a way to relieve stress on the legs. Although it has this effect, it is not the only meaning of kinhin.

When sitting, the legs may become numb or "fall asleep. This does not mean that the circulation is bad, but quite the opposite. There is an old saying in Zen: "*A fire that begins in the toes and consumes your whole body*", this is the meaning of this numbness. The smallest thing - even the legs that go to sleep - is a research topic in our Zen training.

An old question says, *"Can you make your body as soft as a baby's*? When your legs and feet are numb, you'll notice that your ankles are usually flexible. Once, when I was having a private Dokusan with my Zen master, the late Reverend Dr. Soyu Matsuoka-roshi, Archbishop of Soto Zen North America, which consisted of two normal one-hour sessions with Kinhin and no talking - both legs had gone completely to sleep for the final gong. When I crouched, both feet were buzzing in my socks. As I walked toward the altar, the toes of my right foot crawled over the carpet, and bent down to where I was partially standing at the top of my foot. I almost fell! Sensei got me. My foot woke up, but it didn't hurt.

Kinhin is the extension of the stillness of zazen in the action of walking. In your mind, you should strive to eliminate any distinction between the two - they are more alike than different.

There's a famous Zen saying, "Quiet in Action - Quiet in Action". We have this calligraphy of the late Reverend Dr. Soyu Matsuoka-roshi of this expression. It also says, "Silence is Thunder - Mokurai." This is the most essential meaning of walking meditation - it brings the power of meditation into the daily act of walking.

It also symbolizes the fact that the Buddha walks around the bodhi tree after his Enlightenment. So it also represents your "wandering through the world of enlightenment," in the words of Dogen-Zenji, the founder of Soto Zen Buddhism, for the first time.

How to meditate while walking?

The place where the Lord Buddha did meditation walking in Bodhgaya after his Enlightenment still exists to this day. His path was seventeen steps long. These days the Forest Monks tend to make their meditation paths much longer - up to thirty steps long. The beginner may find thirty steps too long because his attention has not yet developed. When you reach the end of the road, your mind may have been "around the world and back. Remember, walking is a stimulating posture, and initially the mind tends to wander a lot. Normally it is best for beginners to start with a shorter path; fifteen steps would be a good length.

If you do an outdoor meditation, look for a secluded place where you won't be distracted or disturbed. It is good to find a slightly closed trail. It may be a distraction to walk in an open area where there is a view, as the mind may be attracted to the landscape. If the path is closed, it tends to lead the mind inwards, towards oneself and towards peace. An enclosed space is especially suitable for speculative personalities who like to think a lot; it helps to calm their minds.

> ### ➤ *Preparing the body and mind*

Once you have chosen a suitable path, stand at one end. Stand up straight. Put your right hand on the left in front of you. Don't walk with your hands behind your back. A meditation teacher who visited the monastery where I was staying once commented when he saw one of the guests walking up and down with his hands behind his back: "He is not walking in meditation; he is going for a walk. By placing your hands in front of you, you create a clear determination to focus the mind on walking meditation, to differentiate it from just walking. ‖

The practice is first to develop samādhi, a Pali word meaning to focus the mind, to develop the mind to one - aiming for gradual degrees of attention and concentration. To focus the mind, one has to be diligent and determined. This requires a degree of both physical and mental composure. You start by composing yourself by holding your hands in front of you. Composing the body helps to compose the mind. Having thus composed the body, one should then remain still and bring consciousness and attention to the body. Then raise your hands together in anjali, a gesture of respect, and with your eyes closed reflect for a few minutes on the qualities of the Buddha, the Dhamma and the Saṅgha.

Behold, you have taken refuge in the Buddha, the Wise One, the One who knows and sees, the Awakened One, the Fully Enlightened One. Reflect in your heart on the qualities of the Buddha for a few minutes. Then remember the

Dhamma-The Truth that you strive to realize on the path of walking meditation.

Finally, bring to mind Saṅgha, especially those fully Enlightened ones who have realized the Truth by cultivating meditation.

Then put your hands down in front of you and make a mental determination of how long you are going to "meditate walking," whether it's half an hour, an hour, or more. No matter how long you decide to walk, stick to it. In this way you are nurturing the mind in that initial stage of meditation with enthusiasm, inspiration and confidence.

The great benefits of active meditation

The Buddha spoke of the five benefits of walking meditation. In the order in which you listed them in this Sutta, they are as follows: walking meditation develops endurance for walking long distances; it is good for striving; it is healthy; it is good for digestion after a meal; and the concentration gained from walking meditation lasts a long time.

The first benefit of walking meditation is that it leads to endurance at walking distances. This was particularly important at the time of the Buddha, when most people traveled on foot. The same Buddha went regularly from place to place, walking up to sixteen kilometers a day. So he recommended that walking meditation be used as a way to develop physical fitness and endurance for long distance walking. The forest monks these days are still wandering; in Thai it is called tudong. They take their bowls and tunics and walk, looking for secluded places to meditate. In preparation for wandering, you progressively increase the amount of meditation as you walk to develop your physical fitness and endurance. Increase the number of hours of meditation walking a day to at least five or six hours.

➤ *The effort*

Effort, especially to overcome drowsiness, is the second benefit. While practicing seated meditation, meditators may fall into quiet states, but if they are "too quiet," they may begin to fall asleep. Without attention and awareness, meditation, even if it feels peaceful, can become clumsiness because it has been overcome by laziness and lethargy. Walking meditation can counteract this trend.

Ajahn Chah used to recommend that once a week we stay up all night, sitting and doing meditation walking all night. We tended to be very sleepy around one or two in the morning, so Ajahn Chah recommended that we do the meditation by walking backwards to overcome sleepiness. You do not fall asleep by walking backwards! Once at Bodhinyana Monastery in Western Australia, I left early one morning, around five o'clock in the morning, to do some walking meditation and saw a layman, who was staying for the Rain Retreat at the monastery, doing meditation walking up and down along the top of the six-foot high wall in front of the monastery. By putting great effort into being attentive to each step, I was overcoming sleepiness by developing a heightened sense of alertness, effort, and zeal.

> ➤ *Health*

The Buddha said that walking meditation leads to good health. This is the third advantage. We are all aware that walking is considered a very good form of exercise. Today, we even hear about power walking. Well, we're talking here about "power meditation," developing walking meditation as both a physical and mental exercise. But to get both benefits, we have to raise awareness of the process of walking, rather than simply walking and letting the mind go away thinking about other things.

> ### *Digestion*

The fourth benefit of walking meditation is that it is good for digestion. This is particularly important for monks who eat one meal a day. After a meal, the blood goes to the stomach and away from the brain. So one can feel sleepy. The forest monks stress that after a meal you have to do a few hours of meditation walking, because walking up and down helps digestion. For lay meditators as well, if you have had a heavy meal, instead of going to bed, go out and do an hour of walking meditation. It will help with physical well-being and provide an opportunity to cultivate the mind.

➢ *Concentration*

The fifth important benefit of walking meditation is that the concentration that arises from walking meditation is maintained for a long time. The walking posture is a relatively coarse or complex meditative posture compared to sitting. While sitting, it is easy to maintain the posture. Our eyes are closed, so there are no visual sensory stimuli, and we are not involved in any body movement.

Therefore, sitting, compared to walking, is a simpler posture in terms of the activities involved. The same is true for standing and lying down, because there is no movement. If one has developed concentration only in the sitting posture, when one rises from that position and begins with body movements such as walking, it is more difficult to maintain that state of concentration. This is because one is moving from a refined state to a coarser state. As we walk there is much more sensory information.

We're looking at where we're going; therefore, there's a visual entrance. There is also a sensory contribution of body movement. Therefore, if we can concentrate the mind as we walk and receive all these sensory stimuli, then when we change from that posture to a simpler one, concentration becomes easier to maintain. That is to say, when we sit down, the force of the mind and the power of that concentration is easily transmitted to this posture. Therefore, walking meditation can help develop the strength and clarity of the mind, and a concentration that can lead to other less active meditation postures.

Walking meditation...

Most people in the West associate meditation with sitting in silence. But traditional Buddhist teachings identify four meditation postures: sitting, walking, standing, and lying down. All four are valid means to cultivate a clear and clear awareness of the present moment. The most common meditation posture after sitting is walking. In meditation centers and monasteries, indoor halls and open-air paths are often built for walking meditation. In meditation retreats, regular walking meditation is an integral part of the program. In practice outside of retreats, some people will include walking as part of their daily meditation practice, for example, ten or twenty minutes of walking before sitting, or walking meditation instead of sitting.

Walking meditation brings a number of

benefits in addition to cultivating mindfulness. It may be a useful way to increase concentration, perhaps in support of sitting practice. When we are tired or lazy, walking can be invigorating. The sensations of walking may be more convincing than the more subtle sensations of breathing while sitting. Walking can be very helpful after a meal, waking from sleep, or after a long period of sitting meditation. In times of strong emotions or stress, walking meditation may be more relaxing than sitting. An additional benefit is that, when done for prolonged periods, walking meditation can increase strength and endurance. People have a variety of attitudes toward walking meditation. Some people take it easily and find it a delight. For many others, the appreciation of this form of meditation takes some time; it is an "acquired taste". However, others see its benefits and do walking meditation even though they don't like it very much.

To do formal meditation while walking, find a trail approximately 30 to 40 feet long, and simply walk from side to side. When you reach the end of your path, stop completely, turn around, stop again, and then start again. Keep your eyes down without looking at anything in particular. Some people find it helpful to keep their eyelids half closed. We get stressed by walking from one side to the other on a single path instead of wandering around because otherwise part of the mind would have to negotiate the path. It takes some mental effort to, say, avoid a chair or walk on a rock. When you walk from one side to the other, you soon know the route and the part of the mind that solves problems can be put to rest.

Walking in a circle is a technique that is sometimes used, but the disadvantage is that the continuity of a circle can hide a wandering mind. Walking back and forth, the small interruption when you stop at the end of your path can help catch your attention if you have wandered. As you walk from side to side, find a rhythm that gives you a sense of ease. I usually advise walking slower than normal, but the pace may vary. Rapid walking can bring a greater sense of ease when you are agitated. Or brisk walking may be appropriate when you are sleepy. When the mind is calm and alert, walking slowly may seem more natural. Your speed may change during a period of walking meditation.

See if you can feel the rhythm that keeps you more intimate and attentive to the physical experience of walking. After you have found a rhythm of tranquility, let your attention settle into the body. Sometimes I find it relaxing to think about letting my body take me for a walk. Once you feel connected to your body, let your attention settle on your feet and lower legs. In sitting meditation, it is common to use the alternating sensations of inhaling and exhaling as an "anchor" that keeps us in the present. In walking meditation, the focus is on the alternate step of the feet.

With your attention on your legs and feet, feel the sensations of each step. Feel your legs and feet tense as you lift your leg. Feel the movement of your leg as it swings in the air. Feel the contact of the foot with the ground. There is no such thing as a "right" experience. You just have to see how the experience feels to you. Every time you notice that the mind has wandered, return it to the sensations of walking feet. Having an idea of the rhythm of the steps can help maintain a continuity of consciousness.

As an aid to staying present, you can wear a silent mental tag for your steps as you walk. The label can be "step, step" or "left, right". Labeling occupies the thinking mind with a rudimentary form of thought, so it is less likely that the mind will move away. Labelling also points the mind towards what you want to observe. Noticing the "step" helps you notice your feet.

If after a while you realize that you are saying "right" for the left foot and "left" for the right foot, you know that your attention has been lost. When walking more slowly, you can try to divide each step into phases and use the traditional "lift, place" labels. To walk very slowly, you can use the "lift, move, and place" labels.

Try to devote your attention to the sensations of walking and let go of everything else. If powerful emotions or thoughts arise and draw your attention away from the sensations of walking, it is often helpful to stop walking and attend to them. When they are no longer convincing, you can return to walking meditation. You may also find something beautiful or interesting that catches your eye as you walk. If you can't let go, stop walking and do the "seek" meditation. Continue walking when you are finished looking.

Some people find that their minds are more active or distracting when walking than when sitting for meditation. This may be because walking is more active and the eyes are open. If so, don't be discouraged and don't think walking is less useful. In fact, it may be more useful to learn to practice with your more everyday mind. You can train your mind to be present every time you walk. Some people choose specific activities in their daily routines to practice walking meditation, such as walking down a hallway at home or at work, or from their car to their workplace.

In our daily lives, we spend more time walking than sitting quietly with our eyes closed. Walking meditation can serve as a powerful bridge between the practice of meditation and daily life, helping us to be more present, attentive and concentrated in ordinary activities. It can reconnect us to the simplicity of being and the vigil that comes from it.

The objects of meditation

The Buddha taught forty different meditation objects, many of which can be used on the path. However, some are more suitable than others. I will discuss here some of these objects of meditation, beginning with those that are most frequently used.

The first method is the awareness of the posture when walking. As you walk, pay full attention to the soles of your feet, to the sensations and feelings that arise and disappear. As you walk, the feeling will change. As the foot rises and comes back into contact with the path, a new feeling arises. Be aware of this sensation on the sole of your foot. Again, as the foot rises, mentally notice the new sensation as it arises. When you lift each foot and place it down, know the sensations you feel. At each new step, certain new feelings are experienced and the old ones cease to exist. These should be known carefully. With each step there is a new feeling experienced: feeling that arises, feeling that disappears; feeling that arises, feeling that disappears.

With this method, we pay attention to the sensation of walking in itself, at each step we take, on the site vedanā (pleasant, unpleasant or neutral sensations). We are aware of any type of vedanā that arises on the soles of the feet. When we stand up, there is a sensation, a sensation, of contact with the ground. This contact may cause pain, heat, or other sensations. We put our attentive attention on these feelings, knowing them completely. When lifting the foot to take a step, the sensation changes as soon as the foot loses contact with the ground. When we put that foot down, again a new sensation arises when the foot comes into contact with the ground. As we walk, feelings constantly change and come up again. We watch closely as this arises and disappears as the soles of the feet rise or touch the ground. In this way we keep all our attention only on the sensations that arise when walking.

Have you ever noticed before the sensations in your feet while walking? They happen every time we walk, but we tend not to notice these subtle things in life. When we walk, our minds tend to be elsewhere. Walking meditation is a way to simplify what we are doing when we are doing it. We are bringing the mind to the "here and now", being "one with the walk to walk". We are simplifying everything, calming the mind by simply knowing the feeling as it comes and goes.

It is important to remember that when you walk you have to keep your eyes down a meter and a half ahead. Don't look around distracted by this or that. Maintain awareness of the sensation on the soles of your feet, and in this way, develop focused attention, and clear knowledge of walking as you walk. How fast should you walk? Ajahn Chah recommended walking naturally, not too slow or too fast. If you walk fast, you may find it very difficult to concentrate on the feeling that the feeling comes and goes. You may have to slow down. On the other hand, some people may need to speed up. You have to find your own rhythm, whatever works for you. You may start slowly at first and then gradually reach your normal walking pace.

If your attention is weak (which means that your mind wanders a lot), then walk very slowly until you can remain in the present moment of every step. Start by establishing attention at the beginning of the road. When you get in the middle of the road, and then mentally ask yourself, "Where is my mind? Is it in the sensation on the soles of my feet? Do I know the contact here and now, at this moment?" If the mind has moved away, then return it to the sensations in the feet again and continue walking. When you reach the end of the road, turn around slowly and restore your attention. Where is the mind? Has it moved away? Do you know the sensation on the soles of your feet? The mind tends to wander to other places chasing thoughts of: anxiety, fear, happiness, sadness, worries, doubts, pleasures, frustrations and all other thoughts that may arise. If attention to the object of meditation is not present, it restores the mind in the simple act of walking, and then begins to walk back to the other end of the path.

When you get to the middle of the road, note again: "Now I am in the middle of the road" and check if the mind is with the object. Then, once you get to the end of the road, mentally write "Where is the mind?". In this way, you walk forward and backward conscious of the feelings that come and go. As you walk, constantly re-establish your attention, attracting the mind backwards, drawing it inwards, making it conscious, knowing the feeling at every moment as it comes and goes.

As you keep an eye on the sensations and feelings on the soles of your feet, you will find that the mind is less distracted. The mind becomes less inclined to go out into the things that are happening around you. You calm down more. The mind becomes calm when it settles. Once the mind is calm and calm, then you will find that walking becomes too coarse an activity for this quality of mind. You'll just want to be still. So stop and stop to allow the mind to experience this calm and tranquility.

Walking implies the mental will to move, and your mind may be too concentrated on the object of meditation to move. Continue standing practice. Meditation has to do with the work of the mind, not with a particular posture. Physical posture is only a convenient means to improve the work of the mind. This calm and tranquility is known as passaddhi; it is one of the factors of the Enlightenment. Concentration and tranquility work together with attention; combined with energy factors, Dhamma research, joy and equanimity, they form the "Seven Factors of Enlightenment". When in meditation the mind is calm, then, due to that calm, a sense of joy, ecstasy and bliss will arise. The Buddha said that the joy of peace is the highest happiness. A concentrated mind experiences that peace, and this peace can be experienced in our lives. Having developed the practice of walking meditation in a formal context, then when we walk in our daily lives by going to the tents, walking from one room to another, we can use this walking activity as meditation. We can be aware simply by walking, simply by being in that process. Our minds can be calm and at peace. This is a way to develop concentration and tranquility in our daily lives.

If while doing sitting meditation, the

mind is reassured with a certain meditation object, then you can use that same object in walking meditation. However, with some subtle objects of meditation, such as breathing, the mind must have achieved a certain degree of stability in that calm first. If the mind is not yet calm and you begin to walk meditating focusing attention on the breath, it will be difficult, as the breath is a very subtle object. It is usually best to start with a coarser object of meditation, such as sensations of feelings that arise in the feet. There are many objects of meditation that transfer well from the posture of sitting to that of walking: for example, the Four of the Divine Abode: Loving Kindness, Compassion, Appreciative Joy, and Equity.

As you go on and on, you develop expansive thoughts based on loving kindness: "May all beings be happy, may all beings be at peace, may all beings be free from all suffering. You can use the walking posture as a complement to sitting, developing meditation on the same object but in a different posture.

Conclusion: Choosing a mantra

If, while walking in meditation, you find that you are falling asleep, activate the mind, instead of calming it, with a mantra to make it more focused and awake. Use a mantra like Buddho, repeating the word quietly over and over again. If the mind still wanders, then it begins to say Buddho very quickly, and walks up and down very fast. As you walk, recite Buddho, Buddho, Buddho, Buddho. In this way, your mind can focus very quickly. Let me tell you a story that illustrates the efficacy of a mantra. When Tan Ajahn Mun, the famous forest meditation master, lived in northern Thailand, the hill tribes of the area knew nothing about the meditation monks. However, the people of the hill tribe are very inquisitive. When they saw him walking up and down his path, they followed him in line. When he turned around at the end of the road, the whole town was standing there.

They had realized that he was walking from side to side with his eyes down and had assumed that he was looking for something. They asked, "What are you looking for, Venerable Lord? Can we help you find him?" He replied skillfully, "I seek Buddha, the Buddha of the heart. You can help me find him by walking up and down your own paths looking for the Buddha. With this simple and beautiful instruction, many of those villagers began to meditate, and Tan Ajahn Mun said they got wonderful results.

> ### *Contemplation of the way things are*

Dhamma research is one of the Illumination Factors. Contemplating the teachings and laws of nature can be employed while walking the path of meditation. This does not mean that one thinks or speculates at random. Rather, it is the constant reflection and contemplation of the Truth, the Dhamma.

➢ *Investigation of impermanence*

For example, one can contemplate Impermanence by observing the process of change, and seeing how all things are subject to change. One develops a clear perception of the emergence and demise of all experience. Life" is a continuous process of arising and dying, and all conditioned experience is subject to this law of nature. In contemplating this Truth, one sees the characteristics of existence. One sees that all things are subject to change. All things are unsatisfactory. All things are not the me. One can investigate these fundamental characteristics of nature on the path of walking meditation.

➢ *Generosity and virtue*

The Buddha continually emphasized the importance of generosity and virtue. On the way one can reflect on one's own virtue or on acts of generosity. Walk up and down and ask yourself, "Today, what acts of kindness have I done?"

A meditation teacher I knew often commented that one of the reasons why meditators can't be calm is because they haven't done enough good during the day. Kindness is a cushion for tranquility, a basis for peace. If we have done acts of kindness during the day - having said a kind word, done a good deed, been generous or compassionate - then the mind will experience joy and ecstasy. These acts of kindness, and the happiness derived from them, will become the conditioning factors for concentration and peace. The powers of kindness and generosity lead to happiness and it is that healthy happiness that forms the basis for concentration and wisdom.

The remembrance of good works is a very appropriate subject of meditation when the mind is restless, agitated, angry, or frustrated. If the mind lacks peace, then remember your past kind actions. This is not for the purpose of building your ego, but for the recognition of the power of goodness and health. Acts of kindness, virtue and generosity bring joy to the mind, and joy is an Enlightenment Factor.

Remember acts of generosity; reflect on the benefits of giving; remember one's own virtue; contemplate the purity of harmlessness, the purity of honesty, the purity of correction in sexual relations, the purity of truthfulness, the purity of not confusing the mind by avoiding intoxicants; all these memories can serve as objects of meditation along the way.

Now yes, I wish you the best in your results, and remember, everything is practical; theory without action is of no use to you.

A big hug, your friend, Jorge!

By the way, when you achieve your

results little by little, I highly recommend you, if you want to learn how to improve your personal and emotional spirituality, my book, on "HOW TO INCREASE YOUR EMOTIONAL AND PERSONAL SPIRITUALITY", is a book that I am sure will help you a lot on your path of "personal, emotional and spiritual growth".

Without further ado, you can find it in the Amazon search engine, like: "How to increase your emotional and personal spirituality" or looking for my name, like: "Jorge O. Chiesa"... Once again I wish you success in your results!

www.ingramcontent.com/pod-product-compliance
Lightning Source LLC
Chambersburg PA
CBHW072025280526
45788CB00007B/2668